Dash Diet Cookbook 2021

-Low Sodium Recipes to Promote Overall Health and Wellness-

[Sebastian Osborne]

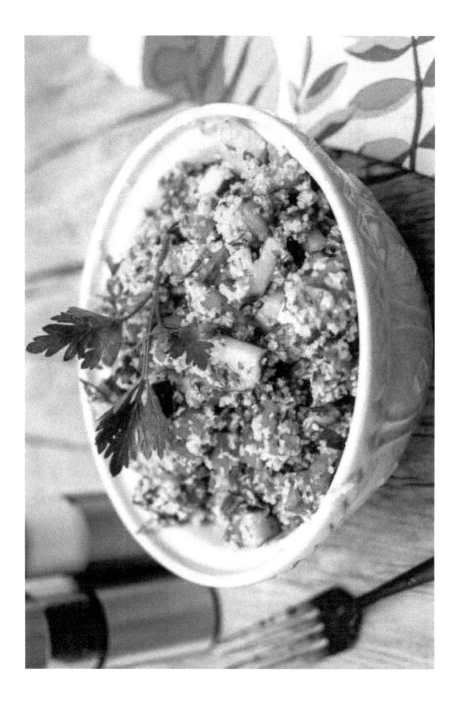

Table Of Content

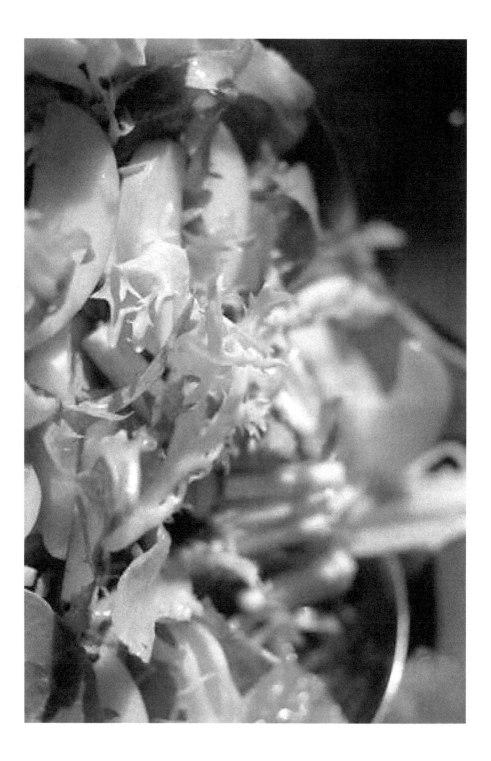

The following Book is reproduced below with the goal of providing information that is as accurate and reliable as possible. Regardless, purchasing this Book can be seen as consent to the fact that both the publisher and the author of this book are in no way experts on the topics discussed within and that any recommendations or suggestions that are made herein are for entertainment purposes only. Professionals should be consulted as needed prior to undertaking any of the action endorsed herein.

This declaration is deemed fair and valid by both the American Bar Association and the Committee of Publishers Association and is legally binding throughout the United States.

Furthermore, the transmission, duplication, or reproduction of any of the following work including specific information will be considered an illegal act irrespective of if it is done electronically or in print. This extends to creating a secondary or tertiary copy of the work or a recorded copy and is only allowed with the express written consent from the Publisher. All additional right reserved.

The information in the following pages is broadly considered a truthful and accurate account of facts and as such, any inattention, use, or misuse of the information in question by the reader will render any resulting actions solely under their purview. There are no scenarios in which the publisher or the original author of this work can be in any fashion deemed liable for any hardship or damages that may befall them after undertaking information described herein.

Additionally, the information in the following pages is intended only for informational purposes and should thus be thought of as universal. As befitting its nature, it is presented without assurance regarding its prolonged validity or interim quality. Trademarks that are mentioned are done without written consent and can in no way be considered an endorsement from the trademark holder.

CHAPTER 1: **BREAKFAST**

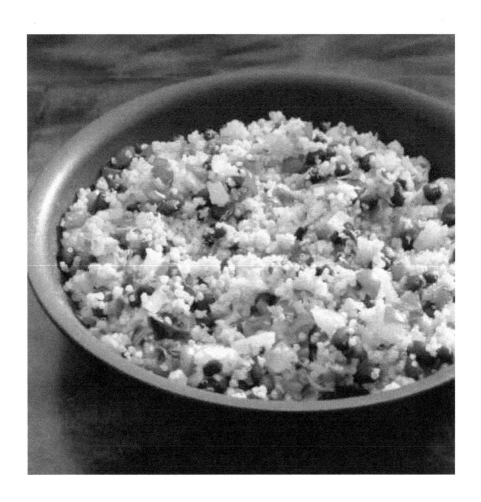

Moming Quinoa

Prep:

5 mins

Cook:

35 mins

Total:

40 mins

Servings:

2

Yield:

2 servings

Ingredients

2 cups chicken broth

2 tablespoons olive oil

2 cloves garlic, minced

1 cup quinoa

1 small onion, diced

1 tablespoon ancho chile powder

salt and pepper to taste

1 tablespoon curry powder

Directions

1

Heat oil in a large skillet over medium heat. Add onion and garlic and cook and stir for 2 minutes; add quinoa and cook and stir until lightly toasted, about 5-6 minutes.

2

Pour broth into the pan and bring to a boil. Reduce heat and add curry and chile powders; cover and simmer until tender, about 25 minutes. Season to taste with salt and pepper.

Nutrition

Per Serving: 473 calories; protein 13.5g; carbohydrates 62.8g; fat 19.8g; sodium 48.2mg

Sweet Millet Congee

Prep:

20 mins

Cook:

3 hrs 15 mins

Total:

3 hrs 35 mins

Servings:

6

Yield:

6 servings

Ingredients

5 cups chicken stock

5 cups water

1 cup white rice

¼ cup apple cider vinegar

½ teaspoon vinegar

1 tablespoon grated fresh ginger

1 teaspoon salt

2 tablespoons fish sauce

2 (6 ounce) fillets lean white fish, sliced

¼ cup sliced Chinese roast pork

2 tablespoons chopped scallions

¼ teaspoon sesame oil

2 tablespoons crushed peanuts

¼ cup pickled Chinese vegetables

½ teaspoon soy sauce

Directions

1

Combine chicken stock, water, rice, 1/4 cup apple cider vinegar, fish sauce, ginger, salt, and sesame oil in a large stockpot; bring to a boil. Reduce heat and simmer until congee has thickened to the consistency of a light porridge, about 3 hours.

2

Stir fish into congee and simmer until cooked through, about 10-12 minutes.

3

Serve congee in bowls topped with pickled vegetables, roast pork, scallions, and peanuts. Drizzle 1/2 teaspoon vinegar and soy sauce over toppings.

Nutrition

Per Serving: 205 calories; protein 15.1g; carbohydrates 28.3g; fat 2.9g; cholesterol 25.4mg; sodium 1430.7mg.

Flax Banana Muffins

Prep:

10 mins

Cook:

20 mins

Total:

30 mins

Servings:

20

Yield:

20 muffins

Ingredients

6 large ripe bananas

1 cup brown sugar

½ cup white sugar

2 eggs

1 ½ cups all-purpose flour

¾ cup salted butter, melted

1 ¼ cups whole wheat flour

2 teaspoons baking soda

2 teaspoons baking powder

½ cup ground flax seeds

Directions

1

Preheat oven to 350 degrees F. Line 2 muffin tins with paper liners.

2

Mash bananas in a bowl. Add brown sugar, butter, white sugar, and eggs; mix well. Add all-purpose flour, whole wheat flour, flax seeds, baking soda, and baking powder. Scoop batter into the prepared tins.

3

Bake in the preheated oven until tops spring back when lightly pressed, about 20-22 minutes.

Nutrition

Per Serving: 240 calories; protein 3.7g; carbohydrates 38.7g; fat 8.9g; cholesterol 36.9mg; sodium 235.5mg.

Multigrain Pancakes

Prep:

10 mins

Cook:

15 mins

Total:

25 mins

Servings:

4

Yield:

4 servings

Ingredients

¼ cup whole wheat flour

¼ cup all-purpose flour

½ teaspoon baking soda

¼ cup rolled oats

¼ cup cornmeal

½ teaspoon salt

1 teaspoon baking powder

½ teaspoon ground cinnamon

2 egg whites

2 tablespoons plain nonfat yogurt

2 tablespoons skim milk

2 teaspoons granular no-calorie sucralose sweetener (e.g., Splenda ®)

2 tablespoons water

Directions

1

In a medium bowl, stir together the whole wheat flour, all-purpose flour, oats, cornmeal, sweetener, salt, baking powder, baking soda and cinnamon. In a separate bowl, whisk together the eggs, yogurt, milk and water. Pour the wet **Ingredients** into the dry, and mix just until moistened.

2

Heat a skillet over medium heat, and coat with cooking spray. Pour about 1/3 cup of batter per pancake onto the skillet. Cook until bubbles begin to form in the center, then flip and cook until browned on the other side.

Nutrition

Per Serving: 120 calories; protein 5.5g; carbohydrates 23.2g; fat 0.7g; cholesterol 0.3mg; sodium 574.8mg.

Light Biscuits

Prep:

15 mins

Cook:

20 mins

Total:

35 mins

Servings:

16

Yield:

16 servings

Ingredients

4 cups all-purpose flour

8 ounces crumbled cooked bacon

1 ½ cups butter, cut into large chunks

1 ¾ cups buttermilk

¼ cup baking powder

Directions

1

Preheat oven to 350 degrees F. Lightly butter 2 muffin tins.

2

Mix flour and baking powder together in a large bowl; cut in butter until mixture resembles coarse crumbs. Stir buttermilk and bacon into flour mixture just until dough holds together.

3

Turn dough onto a floured surface and roll into an even thickness. Fold dough over itself a few times. Cut dough into circles using a cookie or biscuit cutter and arrange circles in the prepared muffin tins.

4

Bake in the preheated oven on the top rack until biscuits are lightly browned, about 23-25 minutes.

Nutrition

Per Serving: 355 calories; protein 9.6g; carbohydrates 26g; fat 23.7g; cholesterol 62.4mg; sodium 746.8mg.

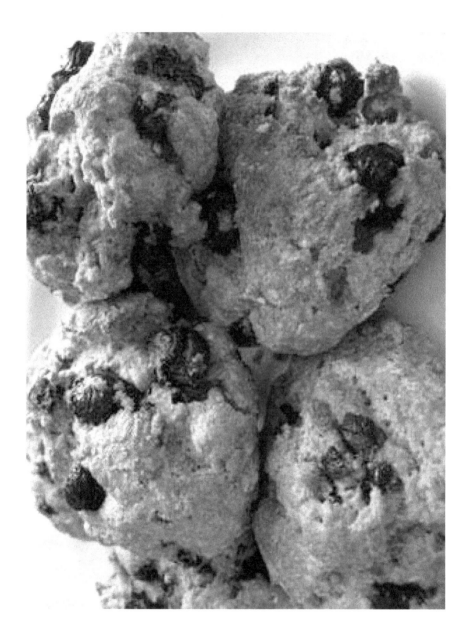

Tofu Smoothie

Prep:

5 mins

Total:

5 mins

Servings:

4

Yield:

4 servings

Ingredients

⅓ (10.75 ounce) package dessert tofu

1 cup orange juice

5 frozen peach slices

1 (8 ounce) container strawberry yogurt

3 frozen strawberries

Directions

1

In a blender, combine tofu, strawberries, peach slices, yogurt and orange juice. Blend until smooth.

Nutrition

Per Serving: 96 calories; protein 3.3g; carbohydrates 19.9g; fat 0.6g; cholesterol 1.2mg; sodium 42.2mg.

Fresh Fruit with Lime Syrup

Prep:

25 mins

Additional:

4 hrs

Total:

4 hrs 25 mins

Servings:

4

Yield:

1 1-quart mold

Ingredients

1 (3 ounce) package lime flavored Jell-O® mix

1 cup cold water

4 rings canned pineapple, drained

1 cup boiling water

½ cup pitted dark sweet cherries, drained

4 pears - peeled, cored and chopped

¼ cup halved seedless red grapes

Directions

1

In a large bowl, dissolve the gelatin in the boiling water. Whisk in the cold water and set aside to cool slightly.

2

Rinse a 1-quart mold in cold water. Stir the pineapple, cherries, grapes and pears into the gelatin and pour into prepared mold. Refrigerate until set, at least four hours.

Nutrition

Per Serving: 242 calories; protein 2.9g; carbohydrates 61.4g; fat 0.3g; sodium 106.8mg.

Mushroom Omelet

Prep:

10 mins

Cook:

25 mins

Total:

35 mins

Servings:

2

Yield:

2 servings

Ingredients

2 tablespoons butter

½ red bell pepper, chopped

½ Bermuda onion, sliced

½ green bell pepper, chopped

½ pound beef tip

½ cup egg substitute

7 baby portobello mushrooms, sliced

Directions

1

Melt butter in a medium saucepan over medium heat. Stir in green bell pepper, red bell pepper, onion and portobello mushrooms. Cook until tender, about 5 minutes.

2

Stir beef into the vegetable mixture, and cook until evenly brown, 5 to 10 minutes.

3

Stir egg beaters into the mixture, and cook 10 minutes, or until firm.

Nutrition

Per Serving: 511 calories; protein 40.2g; carbohydrates 26g; fat 29.5g; cholesterol 104.9mg; sodium 284.2mg.

Toddler Smoothie

Prep:

5 mins

Cook:

8 mins

Additional:

10 mins

Total:

23 mins

Servings:

4

Yield:

4 servings

Ingredients

1 sweet potato

1 banana

¼ cup orange juice

4 strawberries

¼ cup plain Greek yogurt

Directions

1

Prick sweet potato all over with a fork. Microwave on high in 2-minute intervals until tender, turning halfway through, 7 to 10 minutes. Cool sweet potato until easily handled, about 10 minutes.

2

Peel sweet potato and mash coarsely with a fork. Measure out 2 tablespoons and place in a blender. Add banana, Greek yogurt, orange juice, and strawberries; blend until smooth.

Nutrition

Per Serving: 116 calories; protein 2.4g; carbohydrates 24.5g; fat 1.5g; cholesterol 2.8mg; sodium 47.8mg.

Almond Cookies

Servings:

18

Yield:

3 dozen

Ingredients

½ cup butter

1 egg

½ cup white sugar

½ tablespoon ground cinnamon

½ tablespoon ground cloves

½ tablespoon ground nutmeg

⅓ cup finely chopped blanched almonds

2 tablespoons brandy

2 cups all-purpose flour

½ tablespoon lemon zest

Directions

1

Preheat oven to 325 degrees F.

2

Cream the butter until light and fluffy. Add the well beaten egg, almonds, sugar, brandy, spices and flour. Mix until mixture is well combined.

3

On a lightly floured surface roll the mixture to 1/4 inch thick and cut with round cookie cutters dipped in flour. Place cookies onto a parchment lined baking sheet.

4

Bake at 325 degrees F for 9 minutes until lightly browned.

Nutrition

Per Serving: 144 calories; protein 2.5g; carbohydrates 17.1g; fat 7g; cholesterol 23.9mg; sodium 41.8mg.

Asparagus Omelet

Prep:

15 mins

Cook:

10 mins

Total:

25 mins

Servings:

2

Yield:

1 large omelet

Ingredients

3 tablespoons olive oil

¼ cup chopped onion

1 teaspoon garlic salt

¼ cup chopped green pepper

5 large eggs

4 asparagus spears, chopped

2 slices Provolone cheese

1 pound ham steak, cut into small pieces

Directions

1

Heat olive oil in a pan over medium heat; add onion and green pepper. Cook and stir until onion is slightly brown, about 5 minutes. Stir in ham and garlic salt.

2

Beat eggs, asparagus, and milk together with a whisk or a fork in a bowl; pour over ham mixture. Add whole Provolone cheese slices or break them into pieces. Cook until eggs begin to set, about 3 minutes. Gently fold the omelet in half; cook until cheese melts, about 2 minutes.

Nutrition

Per Serving: 739 calories; protein 67.1g; carbohydrates 6.4g; fat 48.8g; cholesterol 531.9mg; sodium 4191.4mg.

Ham and Cheese Omelet

Prep:

15 mins

Cook:

1 hr

Additional:

8 hrs 15 mins

Total:

9 hrs 30 mins

Servings:

6

Yield:

6 servings

Ingredients

1 teaspoon butter for greasing

1 cup cubed Cheddar cheese

1 cup cubed ham

3 cups milk

6 large eggs

12 slices firm bread, discard crusts and cube bread

½ teaspoon ground black pepper

½ teaspoon dried thyme

½ teaspoon salt

Directions

1

Butter bottom and sides of a shallow roasting dish.

2

Layer bread, Cheddar cheese, and ham in prepared roasting dish.

3

Beat milk, eggs, thyme, salt, and black pepper together in a bowl.

4

Pour egg mixture over bread mixture; cover and refrigerate 8 hours or overnight.

5

Preheat oven to 350 degrees F.

6

Bake uncovered egg mixture in the preheated oven until center is set, about 1 hour. Allow to sit and cool for 15 minutes before serving.

Nutrition

Per Serving: 402 calories; protein 23.6g; carbohydrates 32.7g; fat 19.3g; cholesterol 234.5mg; sodium 1095.4mg.

Apple Pancakes

Prep:

15 mins

Cook:

15 mins

Total:

30 mins

Servings:

2

Yield:

2 servings

Ingredients

3 tablespoons butter

1 large apple, cored and sliced

½ cup white sugar, divided

2 teaspoons ground cinnamon

4 eggs

⅓ cup milk

⅓ cup all-purpose flour

1 teaspoon baking powder

1 teaspoon vanilla extract

1 pinch salt

Directions

1

Preheat oven to 400 degrees F (200 degrees C).

2

Melt butter in an oven-safe skillet over medium heat; cook and stir apple slices, about 1/4 cup sugar, and cinnamon in butter until apples are tender, about 5 minutes.

3

Beat eggs, milk, flour, remaining 1/4 cup sugar, baking powder, vanilla extract, and salt in a large bowl until batter is smooth; pour batter evenly over apples.

4

Bake in the preheated oven until golden brown, about 10 minutes. Run a spatula around the edges of the pancake to loosen. Invert skillet over a large plate to serve.

Nutritions

Per Serving: 654 calories; protein 16.6g; carbohydrates 86g; fat 28.4g; cholesterol 421mg; sodium 525.1mg.

Pumpkin Muffins

Prep:

15 mins

Cook:

25 mins

Total:

40 mins

Servings:

40

Yield:

40 muffins

Ingredients

10 eggs

4 cups canned pumpkin puree

2 ⅔ cups vegetable oil

6 cups white sugar

4 ½ teaspoons baking soda

1 teaspoon cream of tartar

1 tablespoon salt

2 teaspoons ground cloves

2 teaspoons ground cinnamon

2 teaspoons ground nutmeg

4 ½ cups matzo cake meal

Directions

1

Preheat oven to 350 degrees F (175 degrees C). Line 40 muffin pan cups with paper muffin liners.

2

Beat eggs, pumpkin puree, and vegetable oil in a large bowl until thoroughly mixed. Stir sugar, baking soda, cream of tartar, salt, cloves, cinnamon, and nutmeg into the egg mixture. Slowly stir matzo cake meal into the batter until combined; pour into prepared muffin cups nearly to the top, as they will not rise much.

3

Bake in the preheated oven until a toothpick inserted into the center comes out clean, 25 to 30 minutes.

Nutritions

Per Serving: 324 calories; protein 3.2g; carbohydrates 44.5g; fat 16g; cholesterol 46.5mg; sodium 394mg.

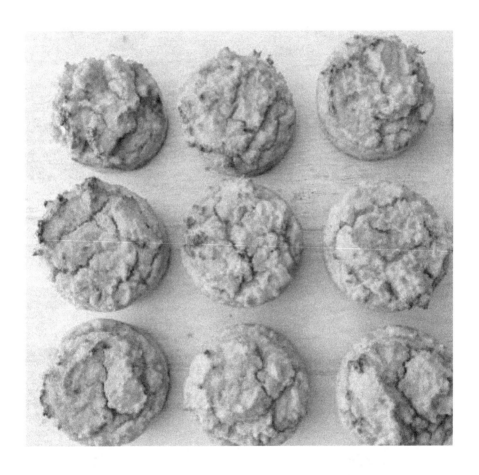

CHAPTER 2: LUNCH

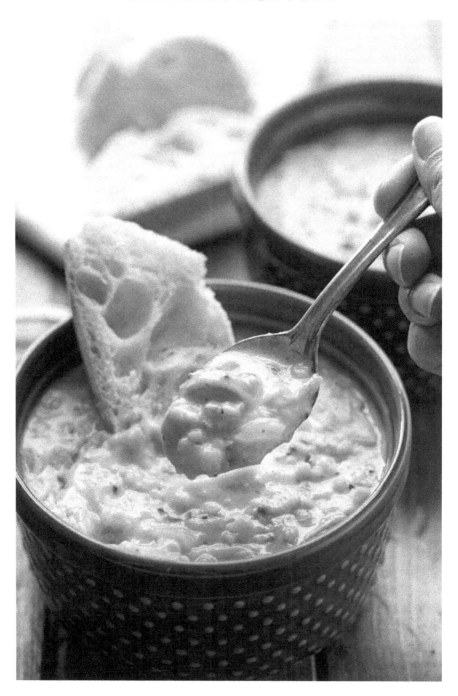

Quinoa Jambalaya

Prep:

10 mins

Cook:

30 mins

Total:

40 mins

Servings:

6

Yield:

6 servings

Ingredients

1 tablespoon vegetable oil

2 cups chicken broth

1 pound kielbasa (Polish) sausage, halved lengthwise and sliced

6 miniature multi-colored sweet peppers, diced

1 teaspoon dried oregano

1 teaspoon dried thyme

½ sweet onion (such as Vidalia®), diced

¼ teaspoon celery salt

1 pinch red pepper flakes

½ teaspoon cayenne pepper

1 cup quinoa

½ cup marinara sauce

Directions

1

Heat oil in a large skillet over medium heat; cook and stir sausage until browned, about 5 minutes. Add onion to sausage; cook and stir until slightly browned, about 5 minutes. Stir sweet pepper, oregano, thyme, cayenne pepper, celery salt, and red pepper flakes into sausage mixture; cook and stir until fragrant, about 2 minutes.

2

Mix quinoa into sausage mixture; cook and stir until quinoa is slightly toasted, about 1 minute. Pour broth and marinara sauce over quinoa mixture. Cover skillet and simmer until quinoa is tender, about 15-17 minutes.

Nutrition

Per Serving: 420 calories; protein 14.7g; carbohydrates 26.1g; fat 27.8g; cholesterol 56.1mg; sodium 1091mg.

Tabbouleh Salad

Prep:

20 mins

Additional:

15 mins

Total:

35 mins

Servings:

8

Yield:

8 servings

Ingredients

3 cups chopped flat-leaf parsley

2 cups finely chopped pineapple

2 cups pomegranate seeds

½ cup fresh lemon juice

½ cup minced onion

¼ cup minced fresh mint leaves

⅔ cup olive oil

salt and ground black pepper to taste

2 cups finely chopped small cucumber

Directions

1

Mix parsley, cucumber, pineapple, pomegranate seeds, onion, and mint in a large bowl. Drizzle olive oil and lemon juice over the salad and toss to coat; season with salt and pepper.

2

Refrigerate salad until chilled, at least 15 minutes.

Nutrition

Per Serving: 231 calories; protein 1.7g; carbohydrates 17.8g; fat 18.4g; sodium 35.3mg.

Chicken with Wild Rice Soup

Prep:

20 mins

Cook:

1 hr 55 mins

Total:

2 hrs 15 mins

Servings:

8

Yield:

8 servings

Ingredients

1 ⅓ cups wild rice

7 cups water

2 tablespoons chicken bouillon granules

1 cup chopped celery

1 cup chopped onion

2 tablespoons vegetable oil

1 cup fresh mushrooms, sliced

¾ cup white wine

¾ teaspoon ground white pepper

½ teaspoon salt

½ cup margarine

¾ cup all-purpose flour

1 (3 pound) whole chicken, cut into pieces

4 cups milk

Directions

1

Cook the wild rice according to package **Directions**, but remove from heat about 15 minutes before it's done. Drain the excess liquid, and set aside.

2

In a stock pot over high heat, combine the chicken and the water. Bring to a boil, and then reduce heat to low. Simmer for 40 minutes, or until chicken is cooked and tender. Remove chicken from the pot, and allow it to cool. Strain the broth from the pot, and reserve for later. When chicken is cool, remove the meat from the bones, cut into bite size pieces, and reserve. Discard the fat and the bones.

3

In the same stock pot over medium heat, saute the celery and onion in the oil for 5 minutes. Add the mushrooms, and cover. Cook for 5 to 10 minutes, stirring occasionally, until everything is tender. Return the broth to the stock pot, and add the partially cooked wild rice. Stir in the bouillon, white pepper and salt; simmer, uncovered, for 15 minutes.

4

Meanwhile, melt margarine in a medium saucepan over medium heat. Stir in the flour until smooth. Whisk in the milk, and continue cooking until mixture is bubbly and thick. Add some of the broth mixture to the milk mixture, continuing to stir, then stir all of the milk mixture into the broth mixture.

5

Mix in the reserved chicken meat and the white wine. Allow this to heat through for about 15 minutes.

Nutrition

Per Serving: 572 calories; protein 33.6g; carbohydrates 38.1g; fat 29.6g; cholesterol 84.5mg; sodium 431.7mg.

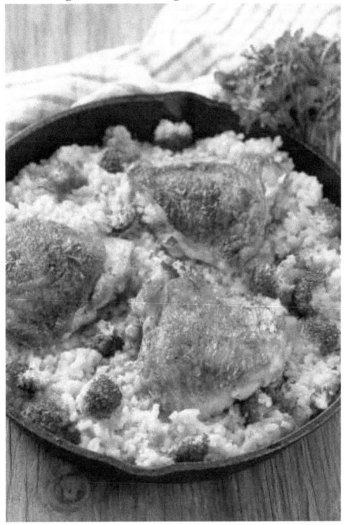

Juicy Chicken

Prep:

20 mins

Cook:

10 mins

Total:

30 mins

Servings:

5

Yield:

5 servings

Ingredients

½ cup soy sauce

1 pound skinless, boneless chicken breast halves - cut into 2 inch pieces

½ cup sherry or white cooking wine

¼ teaspoon ground ginger

1 pinch garlic powder

1 bunch green onions, chopped

½ cup chicken broth

Directions

1

In a small saucepan, combine the soy sauce, sherry, chicken broth, ginger, garlic powder and green onions. Bring to a boil, and immediately remove from heat. Set aside.

2

Preheat your oven's broiler. Thread chicken pieces onto metal or bamboo skewers. Arrange on a broiler pan that has been coated with cooking spray. Spoon 1 or 2 tablespoons of the sauce over each chicken skewer.

3

Place the pan under the broiler, and broil for about 3 minutes, until browned. Remove from the oven, turn over, and spoon more sauce onto each one. Return to the oven until chicken is cooked through and nicely browned.

Nutrition

Per Serving: 152 calories; protein 23.5g; carbohydrates 9.2g; fat 1.2g; cholesterol 52.7mg; sodium 1652.9mg.

Celeriac Salad

Prep:

15 mins

Cook:

30 mins

Total:

45 mins

Servings:

12

Yield:

6 cups

Ingredients

1 celeriac (celery root), peeled and cut into 1/2-inch pieces

⅓ cup heavy cream

3 tablespoons butter

3 potatoes, peeled and cut into 1/2-inch pieces

Directions

1

Place the celeriac cubes into a large pot and cover with salted water. Bring to a boil over high heat, then reduce heat to medium-low, cover, and simmer 12 minutes. Add the potatoes, and continue boiling until the vegetables are very tender, about 15 minutes more. Drain and allow to steam dry for a minute or two.

2

Return the vegetables to the pot, and stir over medium-high heat until liquid is no longer pooling from the vegetables. Remove from the heat,

and pour in the cream and butter. Mash with a potato masher until almost smooth.

Nutrition

Per Serving: 117 calories; protein 2.2g; carbohydrates 15.6g; fat 5.6g; cholesterol 16.7mg; sodium 92.8mg.

Sirloin Soup

Prep:

15 mins

Cook:

15 mins

Total:

30 mins

Servings:

8

Yield:

8 servings

Ingredients

2 tablespoons olive oil
2 pounds top sirloin steak, sliced
½ cup red wine
2 cups chunky pasta sauce
2 cloves garlic, minced
1 onion, thinly sliced

Directions

1

Heat the oil in a 10 inch skillet over medium high heat. Add the onions and saute until tender, about 5 minutes. Add the steak strips, turning so that all sides get browned, about 12 minutes.

2

Add the tomato sauce, garlic and red wine. Reduce heat to low and simmer for 10 to 15 minutes, or until the steak is cooked through.

Nutrition

Per Serving: 276 calories; protein 20g; carbohydrates 10.5g; fat 15.4g; cholesterol 61.7mg; sodium 299.9mg.

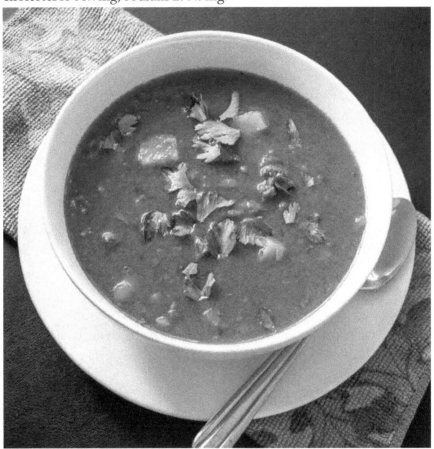

Lasagna Toss

Prep:

15 mins

Cook:

25 mins

Total:

40 mins

Servings:

8

Yield:

8 servings

Ingredients

2 cups uncooked penne pasta

1 cup cottage cheese

1 (26 ounce) jar garlic and onion spaghetti sauce (such as Ragu®
Robusto® Sauteed Onion & Garlic Pasta Sauce)

2 cups shredded mozzarella cheese, divided

1 pound ground Italian sausage

Directions

1

Preheat an oven to 350 degrees F. Grease a 2.5 quart baking dish.

2

Bring a large pot of lightly salted water to a boil. Place pasta in the pot,
cook for 8 to 10 minutes, until tender, and drain.

3

Cook and stir the Italian sausage in a large skillet over medium heat until browned, about 8 to 10 minutes. Drain the fat from the meat, pour the cooked pasta and spaghetti sauce into the skillet, and stir well to combine. Bring the mixture to a boil.

4

Pour half of the hot pasta-sausage mixture into the prepared baking dish, spread with the cottage cheese in an even layer, and sprinkle with half the mozzarella cheese. Spread the remaining pasta mixture over the cheese, and top with the remaining mozzarella cheese.

5

Cover and bake in the preheated oven for about 25 minutes, until the casserole is hot and the cheese is melted and bubbling. Let it stand 5 minutes to firm up before serving.

Nutrition

Per Serving: 386 calories; protein 22.1g; carbohydrates 29.6g; fat 19.3g; cholesterol 46.4mg; sodium 1134.6mg.

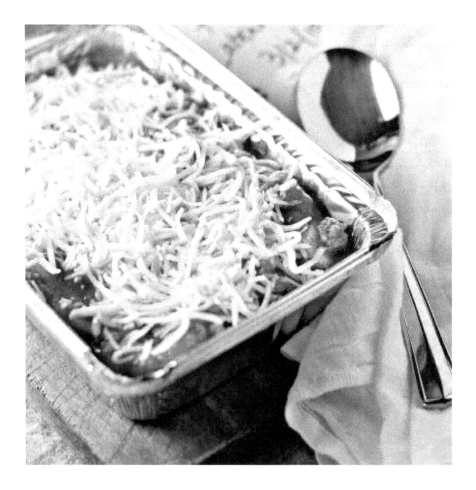

Veggie Burgers

Prep:

15 mins

Cook:

20 mins

Total:

35 mins

Servings:

4

Yield:

4 patties

Ingredients

1 (16 ounce) can black beans, drained and rinsed

½ cup bread crumbs

½ green bell pepper, cut into 2 inch pieces

½ onion, cut into wedges

1 egg

1 tablespoon chili powder

1 tablespoon cumin

1 teaspoon Thai chili sauce or hot sauce

3 cloves garlic, peeled

Directions

   1

If grilling, preheat an outdoor grill for high heat, and lightly oil a sheet of aluminum foil. If baking, preheat oven to 375 degrees F, and lightly oil a baking sheet.

2

In a medium bowl, mash black beans with a fork until thick and pasty.

3

In a food processor, finely chop bell pepper, onion, and garlic. Then stir into mashed beans.

4

In a small bowl, stir together egg, chili powder, cumin, and chili sauce.

5

Stir the egg mixture into the mashed beans. Mix in bread crumbs until the mixture is sticky and holds together. Divide mixture into four patties.

6

If grilling, place patties on foil, and grill about 8 minutes on each side. If baking, place patties on baking sheet, and bake about 10 minutes on each side.

Nutrition

Per Serving: 198 calories; protein 11.2g; carbohydrates 33.1g; fat 3g; cholesterol 46.5mg; sodium 607.3mg.

Farro Salad

Prep:

20 mins

Cook:

30 mins

Additional:

15 mins

Total:

1 hr 5 mins

Servings:

6

Yield:

6 servings

Ingredients

3 cups chicken stock

1 cup uncooked farro

½ cup crumbled feta cheese

1 green bell pepper, finely chopped

½ cup diced sun-dried tomatoes

½ small red onion, finely chopped

¼ cup chopped fresh parsley

1 roasted red pepper, diced

Greek Vinaigrette:

3 tablespoons olive oil

1 tablespoon red wine vinegar

¼ teaspoon dried oregano

1 pinch salt

1 tablespoon lemon juice

1 pinch ground black pepper
1 pinch garlic powder

Directions

1

Bring chicken stock and farro to a boil in a saucepan. Reduce heat to medium-low, cover, and simmer until tender but still chewy, 25 to 30 minutes. Transfer farro to a large bowl and let cool, at least 15 minutes.

2

Add peppers, sun-dried tomatoes, onion, and parsley to the bowl of farro. Toss together and stir in feta cheese.

3

Mix olive oil, lemon juice, vinegar, oregano, salt, garlic powder, and black pepper together. Toss vinaigrette with the salad. Serve cooled.

Nutrition

Per Serving: 223 calories; protein 6.7g; carbohydrates 29.1g; fat 10.9g; cholesterol 11.5mg; sodium 660.4mg.

Basic Vinaigrette

Prep:

5 mins

Total:

5 mins

Servings:

8

Yield:

1 cup

Ingredients

½ cup red wine vinegar
1 clove crushed garlic
2 teaspoons white sugar
½ cup vegetable oil
2 teaspoons salt

Directions

1

In a jar with a tight fitting lid, combine vinegar, oil, garlic, sugar, and salt. Shake well.

Nutrition

Per Serving: 130 calories; carbohydrates 2.2g; fat 13.8g; sodium 581.4mg.

Chipotle Dip

Prep:

10 mins

Cook:

5 mins

Total:

15 mins

Servings:

8

Yield:

8 servings

Ingredients

½ cup paleo mayonnaise

½ cup chopped fresh cilantro

1 clove garlic

2 tablespoons olive oil

1 lime, juiced

2 chipotle peppers in adobo sauce

Directions

1

Combine paleo mayonnaise, chipotle peppers, fresh cilantro, olive oil, lime juice, and garlic in a food processor or blender. Pulse or blend mixture until smooth and well combined, about 1 minute.

Nutrition

Per Serving: 133 calories; protein 0.2g; carbohydrates 1.3g; fat 14.4g; cholesterol 5.2mg; sodium 95.5mg.

Orzo with Feta

Prep:

30 mins

Cook:

10 mins

Additional:

1 hr

Total:

1 hr 40 mins

Servings:

6

Yield:

6 servings

Ingredients

¼ cup olive oil

2 cloves garlic, minced

½ cup fresh lemon juice

½ cup pitted kalamata olives, chopped

1 red bell pepper, chopped

1 red onion, chopped

1 teaspoon finely chopped fresh oregano

2 ripe tomatoes, seeded and diced

½ pound dried orzo pasta

1 cup chopped fresh parsley

1 (8 ounce) package crumbled feta cheese

Directions

1

Stir together olive oil, lemon juice, olives, tomatoes, red pepper, red onion, garlic, oregano, and feta cheese in a large bowl. Let stand at room temperature for 1 hour.

2

Bring a large pot of lightly salted water to a boil. Add the orzo and cook for 8 to 10 minutes or until al dente; drain and toss the tomato mixture. Sprinkle with chopped parsley to serve.

Nutrition

Per Serving: 381 calories; protein 12g; carbohydrates 38.4g; fat 20.8g; cholesterol 33.7mg; sodium 617.6mg.

Leeks Soup

Prep:

20 mins

Cook:

40 mins

Total:

1 hr

Servings:

4

Yield:

4 servings

Ingredients

2 tablespoons butter

3 leeks (white and pale green parts only), thinly sliced

1 clove garlic, minced

1 (32 fluid ounce) container chicken stock

1 ½ cups thinly sliced carrots

2 stalks celery, thinly sliced

1 teaspoon curry powder

½ teaspoon ground turmeric

½ teaspoon ground ginger

⅛ teaspoon ground black pepper

1 pinch red pepper flakes

1 ½ (12 ounce) cans light coconut milk

Directions

1

Melt butter in a stockpot over medium heat. Cook and stir leeks and garlic in melted butter until tender, about 5 minutes.

2

Stir chicken stock, carrots, celery, curry powder, turmeric, ginger, black pepper, and red pepper flakes with the leeks and garlic; bring to a boil, reduce heat to medium-low, cover the pot, and simmer the mixture until vegetables are tender, about 30 minutes.

3

Pour coconut milk into the soup and stir; cook just until hot, 1 to 2 minutes.

Nutritions

Per Serving: 257 calories; protein 3.6g; carbohydrates 18.9g; fat 18.9g; cholesterol 16mg; sodium 798.2mg.

Salmon Wrap

Prep:

30 mins

Total:

30 mins

Servings:

2

Yield:

2 wraps

Ingredients

2 green onions, chopped

⅓ cup thinly julienned daikon radish

⅓ cup chopped cucumber

1 tablespoon rice wine vinegar

1 tablespoon soy sauce

¼ teaspoon wasabi paste

⅛ teaspoon ground ginger

2 (12 inch) flour tortillas

1 cup cooked white rice

⅔ cup canned salmon, drained

2 teaspoons sesame seeds

Directions

1

Toss together the green onion, daikon radish, and cucumber in a small bowl. In a separate bowl, whisk together the rice wine vinegar, soy sauce, wasabi paste, and ground ginger.

2

Lay to two tortillas onto a flat surface. Divide the rice and place in the center of each tortilla. Top each portion of rice with half of the salmon and half of the vegetable mixture. Drizzle half of the soy sauce mixture over each portion of vegetables. Sprinkle each with 1 teaspoon sesame seeds. Wrap the edges of the tortillas around the filling completely to serve.

Nutritions

Per Serving: 891 calories; protein 39.3g; carbohydrates 138.5g; fat 18g; cholesterol 40.5mg; sodium 1551.3mg.

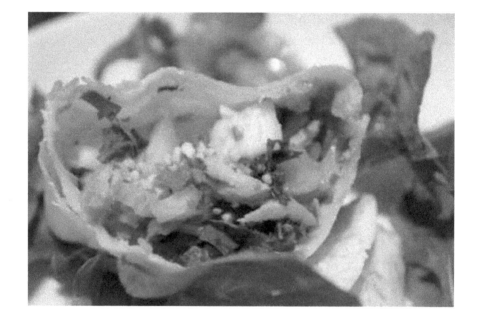

CHAPTER 3: DINNER

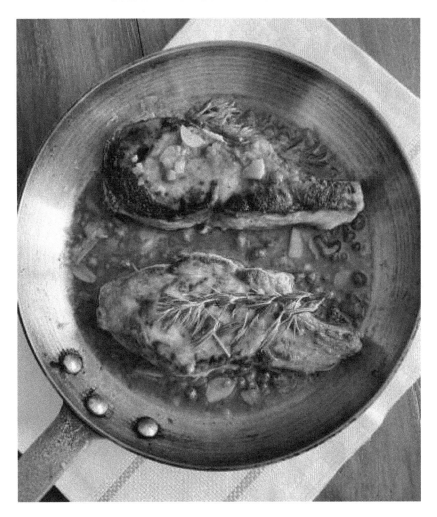

Pork Chops with Black Beans

Prep:

5 mins

Cook:

25 mins

Total:

30 mins

Servings:

4

Yield:

4 servings

Ingredients

4 bone-in pork chops
1 tablespoon chopped fresh cilantro
ground black pepper to taste
1 (15 ounce) can black beans, with liquid
1 cup salsa
1 tablespoon olive oil

Directions

1

Season pork chops with pepper.

2

Heat oil in a large skillet over medium-high heat. Cook pork chops in hot oil until browned, 3 to 5 minutes per side.

3

Pour beans and salsa over pork chops and season with cilantro. Bring to a boil, reduce heat to medium-low, cover the skillet, and simmer until pork chops are cooked no longer pink in the center, 20 to 40 minutes. An instant-read thermometer inserted into the center should read 145 degrees F.

Nutrition

Per Serving: 392 calories; protein 33.8g; carbohydrates 21.8g; fat 18.7g; cholesterol 72.1mg; sodium 836.5mg.

Pantry Puttanesca

Prep:

5 mins

Cook:

16 mins

Total:

21 mins

Servings:

4

Yield:

4 servings

Ingredients

⅓ cup olive oil

¼ cup capers, chopped

3 cloves garlic, minced

¼ teaspoon crushed red pepper flakes

1 teaspoon dried oregano

2 (15 ounce) cans diced tomatoes, drained.

1 (8 ounce) package spaghetti

½ cup chopped pitted kalamata olives

3 anchovy fillets, chopped

Directions

1

Fill a large pot with water. Bring to a rolling boil over high heat.

2

As the water heats, pour the olive oil into a cold skillet and stir in the garlic. Turn heat to medium-low and cook and stir until the garlic is fragrant and begins to turn a golden color, 1 to 2 minutes. Stir in the red pepper flakes, oregano, and anchovies. Cook until anchovies begin to break down, about 2 minutes.

3

Pour tomatoes into skillet, turn heat to medium-high, and bring sauce to a simmer. Use the back of a spoon to break down tomatoes as they cook. Simmer until sauce is reduced and combined, about 12 minutes.

4

Meanwhile, cook the pasta in the boiling water. Drain when still very firm to the bite, about 10 minutes. Reserve 1/2 cup pasta water.

5

Stir the olives and capers into the sauce; add pasta and toss to combine.

6

Toss pasta in sauce until pasta is cooked through and well coated with sauce, about 1 minute. If sauce becomes too thick, stir in some of the reserved pasta water to thin.

Nutrition
Per Serving: 463 calories; protein 10.5g; carbohydrates 53.3g; fat 24g; cholesterol 2.5mg; sodium 944.5mg.

Sloppy Toms

Prep:

30 mins

Cook:

1 hr 15 mins

Total:

1 hr 45 mins

Servings:

25

Yield:

5 pints

Ingredients

5 cups chopped green tomatoes

5 (1 pint) canning jars with lids and rings

2 tablespoons finely chopped crystallized ginger

1 ½ cups chopped onion

2 ¼ cups packed brown sugar

½ teaspoon salt

1 ¾ cups apple cider vinegar

1 ½ cups golden raisins

1 ½ tablespoons pickling spice

1 ½ teaspoons chili powder

1 tablespoon brown mustard seed

4 cups fresh tomatillos, husked, rinsed, and chopped

Directions

1

Place the green tomatoes, tomatillos, raisins, onion, brown sugar, salt, apple cider vinegar, pickling spice, chili powder, crystallized ginger, and brown mustard seed into a large pot over medium heat. Bring to a boil, and stir until the brown sugar has dissolved. Reduce heat, and simmer the chutney until thickened, 1 to 2 hours, stirring occasionally to keep chutney from burning on the bottom.

2

Sterilize the jars and lids in boiling water for at least 5 minutes. Pack the chutney into the hot, sterilized jars, filling the jars to within 1/4 inch of the top. Run a knife or a thin spatula around the insides of the jars after they have been filled to remove any air bubbles. Wipe the rims of the jars with a moist paper towel to remove any food residue. Top with lids, and screw on rings.

3

Place a rack in the bottom of a large stockpot and fill halfway with water. Bring to a boil over high heat, then carefully lower the jars into the pot using a holder. Leave a 2 inch space between the jars. Pour in more boiling water if necessary until the water level is at least 1 inch above the tops of the jars. Bring the water to a full boil, cover the pot, and process for 15 to 20 minutes, or the time recommended by your county Extension office.

4

Remove the jars from the stockpot and place onto a cloth-covered or wood surface, several inches apart, until cool. Once cool, press the top of each lid with a finger, ensuring that the seal is tight (lid does not move up or down at all). Store in a cool, dark area. Any uncanned chutney can be refrigerated or frozen.

Nutrition

Per Serving: 135 calories; protein 1.3g; carbohydrates 32.8g; fat 0.6g; sodium 61.2mg.

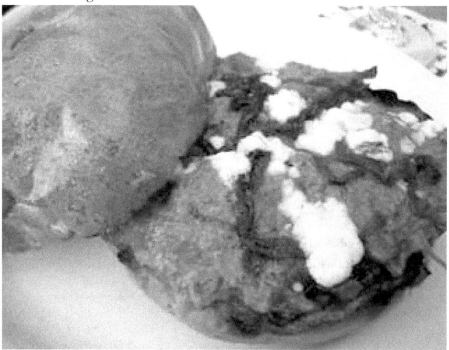

Fettuccine with Basil

Servings:

2

Yield:

2 servings

Ingredients

¾ cup chopped fresh basil
2 ½ tablespoons all-purpose flour
1 egg
1 teaspoon olive oil
2 tablespoons water
1 ½ cups all-purpose flour

Directions

1

Using a food processor, process basil leaves until chopped very fine.
Add 1 1/2 cups of flour and pulse two or three times, or until
combined. Add egg, 1 teaspoon oil, and the water until dough forms a
ball shape. If dough seems dry, add a bit more water. Wrap dough in a
piece of plastic wrap which has been coated in a few drops of olive oil.
Refrigerate dough for 2 hours.

2

Remove dough from refrigerator, and cut into 6 equal size portions.
Run pasta though pasta machine, or roll with rolling pin to desired
thickness. Use the additional flour to coat pasta while rolling.

3

Allow pasta to dry for one hour prior to cooking.

4

Cook in a large pot of boiling water until al dente. This should take only a 3 to 6 minutes, depending on the thickness of the pasta.

Nutrition

Per Serving: 437 calories; protein 14.3g; carbohydrates 79.6g; fat 6g; cholesterol 93mg; sodium 38.2mg.

Pasta Soup

Prep:

15 mins

Cook:

25 mins

Total:

40 mins

Servings:

4

Yield:

4 servings

Ingredients

¾ pound Italian sausage

2 tablespoons chopped fresh basil

½ cup diced onion

6 cups chicken broth

¼ teaspoon ground black pepper

5 ounces farfalle pasta

½ teaspoon Italian seasoning

½ teaspoon salt, or to taste

½ cup ricotta cheese

½ cup shredded mozzarella cheese

¼ cup freshly grated Parmesan cheese

1 (15 ounce) can diced tomatoes with basil, garlic, and oregano

Directions

1

Cook Italian sausage and onion in a skillet over medium-high heat until sausage is browned and crumbly and onion is soft and translucent, about 7 minutes.

2

Mix in chicken broth, diced tomatoes, pasta, Italian seasoning, salt, and pepper. Bring to a boil. Reduce heat and simmer until pasta is tender, stirring occasionally, about 10 minutes. Add ricotta cheese and cook until ricotta is fully incorporated, 2 to 3 minutes more.

3

Top each serving with 2 tablespoons mozzarella cheese, 1 tablespoon Parmesan cheese, and 1/2 tablespoon fresh basil.

Nutrition

Per Serving: 482 calories; protein 27.4g; carbohydrates 37.5g; fat 23.7g; cholesterol 64.7mg; sodium 3111.4mg.

Sirloin Marinara

Prep:

15 mins

Cook:

15 mins

Total:

30 mins

Servings:

8

Yield:

8 servings

Ingredients

2 tablespoons olive oil

2 pounds top sirloin steak, sliced

2 cups chunky pasta sauce

1 onion, thinly sliced

½ cup red wine

2 cloves garlic, minced

Directions

1

Heat the oil in a 10 inch skillet over medium high heat. Add the onions and saute until tender, about 5 minutes. Add the steak strips, turning so that all sides get browned, about 10 minutes.

2

Add the tomato sauce, garlic and red wine. Reduce heat to low and simmer for 11 to 15 minutes, or until the steak is cooked through.

Nutrition

Per Serving: 276 calories; protein 20g; carbohydrates 10.5g; fat 15.4g; cholesterol 61.7mg; sodium 299.9mg.

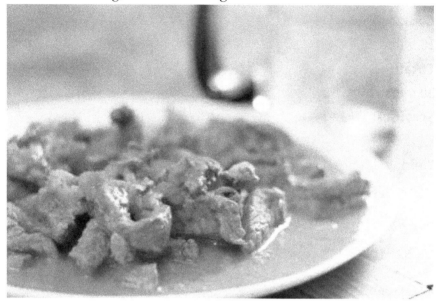

Beef Tacos

Prep:

15 mins

Additional:

30 mins

Total:

45 mins

Servings:

6

Yield:

6 servings

Ingredients

PAM® Original No-Stick Cooking Spray

1 pound ground chuck beef (80% lean)

2 cups frozen Southwest mixed vegetables (corn, black beans, red peppers)

1 (10 ounce) can Ro*Tel® Original Diced Tomatoes & Green Chilies, undrained

1 (10 ounce) can red enchilada sauce

6 ounces dry extra-wide egg noodles, uncooked

1 ¼ cups water

¼ cup thinly sliced green onions

1 teaspoon Sour cream

1 ¼ cups shredded Mexican blend cheese

Directions

1

Preheat oven to 400 degrees F.

2

Spray 13x9-inch glass baking dish with cooking spray. Place uncooked noodles in baking dish.

3

Heat large skillet over medium-high heat. Add beef; cook 6-7 minutes or until crumbled and no longer pink. Drain. Add vegetables, undrained tomatoes, enchilada sauce and water to skillet; stir. Bring to a boil. Pour mixture over noodles.

4

Cover dish tightly with foil; bake 15 minutes. Stir; sprinkle with cheese and cover with foil. Bake 10 minutes more or until noodles are tender. Sprinkle with green onions. Serve with sour cream, if desired.

Nutrition

Per Serving: 474 calories; protein 25.8g; carbohydrates 30.9g; fat 27g; cholesterol 107.6mg; sodium 656.6mg.

South Western Steak

Prep:

15 mins

Cook:

15 mins

Additional:

20 mins

Total:

50 mins

Servings:

4

Yield:

4 servings

Ingredients

2 (1 pound) flat iron steaks, at room temperature

1 tablespoon smoked paprika

1 teaspoon dry beef bouillon powder

5 tablespoons olive oil

3 tablespoons minced garlic

2 tablespoons chili powder

1 tablespoon balsamic vinegar

1 tablespoon lime juice

½ teaspoon dried cilantro

¼ cup finely chopped onion

1 tablespoon molasses

1 tablespoon onion powder

1 teaspoon ground cumin

¼ teaspoon ground black pepper

1 pinch dried rubbed sage

Directions

1

Rub steaks all over with beef bouillon powder.

2

Preheat an outdoor grill for medium-high heat and lightly oil the grate.

3

Whisk olive oil, onion, garlic, chili powder, balsamic vinegar, lime juice, molasses, paprika, onion powder, cumin, cilantro, black pepper, and sage together in a shallow baking dish until marinade is thick and well-combined. Place steaks in marinade and turn to coat completely. Cover the dish with plastic wrap and let stand at room temperature to marinate meat, about 15 minutes.

4

Cook the steaks on the preheated grill, basting frequently with marinade, until steaks start to firm and are reddish-pink and juicy in the center, 6 to 7 minutes per side. An instant-read thermometer inserted into the center should read 130 degrees F. Remove steaks to a plate and let rest for 3 minutes before slicing.

Nutrition

Per Serving: 634 calories; protein 48.3g; carbohydrates 12.8g; fat 44.2g; cholesterol 154.9mg; sodium 303.4mg.

Chives Chicken

Prep:

15 mins

Cook:

1 hr

Total:

1 hr 15 mins

Servings:

4

Yield:

4 servings

Ingredients

1 head garlic

1 (8 ounce) package egg noodles

1 cup chicken broth

¼ teaspoon salt

¼ teaspoon ground black pepper

2 teaspoons olive oil

1 lemon, zested and juiced

4 skinless, boneless chicken breast halves

4 tablespoons butter

⅓ cup chopped fresh chives

2 tablespoons all-purpose flour

Directions

1

Preheat oven to 400 degrees F. Wrap the garlic head in foil, and bake 30 minutes, until cloves are soft. Remove from heat, and cool enough to handle.

2

Bring a large pot of lightly salted water to a boil. Add egg noodles and cook for 7 minutes or until al dente; drain.

3

Slice off the top of the garlic head, and squeeze the softened cloves into a medium bowl. Mix in the chicken broth, lemon zest, lemon juice, salt, and pepper.

4

Heat the olive oil in a skillet over medium heat. Lightly coat the chicken breast halves with flour, and cook in the skillet about 10 minutes on each side, until lightly browned. Set chicken aside, retaining skillet juices. Stir in the garlic mixture, and bring to a boil. Reduce heat, and return chicken to the skillet. Continue cooking the chicken about 5 minutes on each side, until no longer pink and juices run clear. Remove chicken, and arrange on plates over the egg noodles.

5

Mix the butter into the garlic sauce mixture in the skillet until melted, and stir in the chives. Spoon the sauce over the chicken and egg noodles to serve.

Nutrition

Per Serving: 482 calories; protein 31.4g; carbohydrates 46.3g; fat 19.6g; cholesterol 133.5mg; sodium 578.3mg.

Balsamic Salmon

Prep:

10 mins

Cook:

20 mins

Total:

30 mins

Servings:

8

Yield:

8 servings

Ingredients

8 salmon fillets, 3/4-inch thick

Ground black pepper

1 ¾ cups Swanson® Chicken Stock

3 tablespoons balsamic vinegar

1 ½ tablespoons cornstarch

3 tablespoons olive oil

1 tablespoon orange juice

1 teaspoon grated orange zest

Orange slices

1 tablespoon packed brown sugar

Directions

1

Season the salmon with the black pepper. Place the salmon into a 2-quart shallow baking dish. Drizzle with the olive oil. Bake at 350 degrees F for 15 minutes or until the salmon flakes easily when tested with a fork.

2

Heat the stock, vinegar, cornstarch, orange juice, brown sugar and orange zest in a 2-quart saucepan over medium-high heat to a boil. Cook and stir until the mixture boils and thickens.

3

Serve the salmon with the citrus sauce. Garnish with the orange slices.

Nutrition

Per Serving: 253 calories; protein 20.8g; carbohydrates 4.9g; fat 16.2g; cholesterol 56.5mg; sodium 168.5mg.

Tortellini with Pesto

Prep:

10 mins

Cook:

30 mins

Total:

40 mins

Servings:

6

Yield:

6 servings

Ingredients

2 tablespoons olive oil

1 ½ pounds chicken breast, cubed

1 cup Parmesan cheese, divided

½ cup chicken broth

½ cup heavy cream

1 cup baby spinach

½ cup prepared pesto

½ cup cherry tomatoes, halved

1 (16 ounce) package refrigerated cheese tortellini

salt and ground black pepper to taste

Directions

1

Heat olive oil in a large skillet over medium-high heat. Add chicken to the skillet and season with salt and pepper. Saute until chicken is cooked through and has browned, 6 to 10 minutes. Remove from skillet and transfer to a bowl; cover to keep warm. Set aside.

2

Deglaze pan with chicken broth over medium heat, scraping up any browned bits. Stir in pesto and heavy cream. Cook until thickened, 3 to 5 minutes. Mix in 1/2 cup Parmesan cheese and stir until melted. Add in spinach and tomatoes. Cook until spinach begins to wilt, 3 to 5 minutes.

3

Add tortellini and cooked chicken and continue cooking until bubbly and hot, 5 to 10 minutes. Sprinkle with remaining 1/2 cup of Parmesan cheese and serve.

Nutrition

Per Serving: 634 calories; protein 43.5g; carbohydrates 38g; fat 34.5g; cholesterol 143.4mg; sodium 834.8mg.

Green Pea and Ham Salad

Prep:

10 mins

Additional:

2 hrs

Total:

2 hrs 10 mins

Servings:

6

Yield:

6 servings

Ingredients

1 (10 ounce) package frozen peas, thawed and drained

1 ½ teaspoons mustard

1 cup shredded Cheddar cheese

¾ cup mayonnaise

2 tablespoons onion, chopped

2 cups cubed fully cooked ham

Directions

1

Mix peas, ham, Cheddar cheese, mayonnaise, onion, and Dijon mustard in a large bowl. Cover and refrigerate at least 2 hours before serving.

Nutrition

Per Serving: 423 calories; protein 15.8g; carbohydrates 8g; fat 36.6g; cholesterol 55.4mg; sodium 918.7mg.

Grilled Salmon With Pesto Crust

Prep:

15 mins

Cook:

20 mins

Total:

35 mins

Servings:

4

Yield:

4 servings

Ingredients

¼ cup pine nuts

¼ cup grated Parmesan cheese

1 clove garlic, minced

3 tablespoons extra-virgin olive oil

1 pound salmon fillet

½ cup coarsely chopped fresh basil

salt and freshly ground black pepper to taste

Directions

1

Heat a small skillet over medium heat; cook and stir pine nuts in the hot skillet until fragrant and toasted, about 5 minutes.

2

Blend basil, Parmesan cheese, toasted pine nuts, and garlic in a blender until a thick paste forms. Gradually stream olive oil into blender and continue blending until desired consistency of pesto is reached; season with salt and pepper.

3

Preheat an outdoor grill for medium-high heat and lightly oil the grate. Season both sides of salmon with salt and pepper.

4

Place salmon, skin-side down, onto grill grates; close grill and cook until salmon is about 2/3 done, 8 to 15 minutes. Remove salmon from grill using a spatula and transfer to a baking sheet, skin-side down. Spread pesto evenly over the salmon. Save extra pesto for another use if there are leftovers.

5

Set oven rack about 6 inches from the heat source and preheat the oven's broiler.

6

Broil salmon until fish flakes easily with a fork and pesto is bubbling, about 5 minutes.

Nutrition
Per Serving: 354 calories; protein 28.3g; carbohydrates 1.8g; fat 25.6g; cholesterol 81.4mg; sodium 174.3mg.

Beef Soup

Prep:

10 mins

Cook:

30 mins

Total:

40 mins

Servings:

6

Yield:

6 servings

Ingredients

1 pound lean ground beef

48 ounces tomato-vegetable juice cocktail

2 (16 ounce) packages frozen mixed vegetables

Directions

1

Place ground beef in a Dutch oven or slow cooker. Cook over medium-high heat until evenly brown. Drain excess fat, and crumble. Add juice cocktail and mixed vegetables.

2

In a Dutch oven, simmer for 30 minutes.

3

In a slow cooker, cook 1 hour on High. Then reduce heat to Low and simmer 6 to 8 hours.

Nutritions

Per Serving: 343 calories; protein 20.3g; carbohydrates 29.6g; fat 16.4g; cholesterol 56.8mg; sodium 694.9mg.

CHAPTER 4: SNACK & APPETIZER

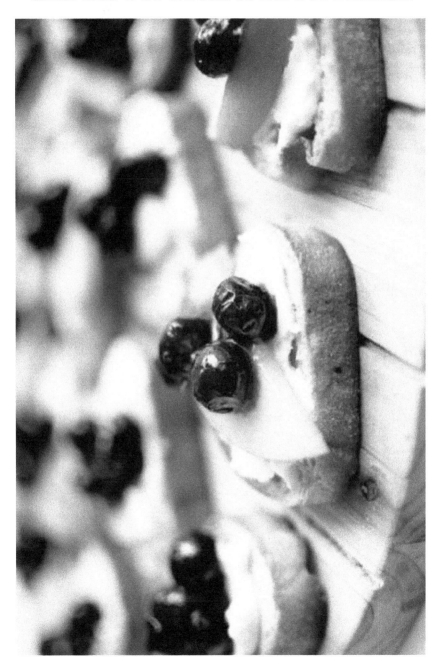

Shrimp Ceviche

Prep:

15 mins

Cook:

5 mins

Additional:

20 mins

Total:

40 mins

Servings:

4

Yield:

4 servings

Ingredients

1 cucumber, diced

½ pound raw shrimp, peeled and deveined

2 Roma tomatoes, diced

1 ½ teaspoons salt, divided

½ medium red onion, diced

2 serrano peppers, seeded and deveined

¼ cup chopped cilantro

6 medium limes, divided

½ teaspoon ground black pepper to taste

Directions

1

Combine cucumber, tomatoes, red onion, serrano peppers, and cilantro in a bowl. Add 1 teaspoon salt and squeeze 1 lime. Gently mix and set aside.

2

Squeeze the remaining limes into another bowl. Add remaining salt and pepper.

3

Bring a 1- to 2-quart pot of water to a boil. Place shrimp into the boiling water for 45 seconds. Quickly remove from the water using a strainer.

4

Chop the partially cooked shrimp into small pieces and add to the bowl with the seasoned lime mixture. Let sit for 20 minutes. Combine with the cucumber mixture and top with avocados.

Nutrition

Per Serving: 163 calories; protein 11.7g; carbohydrates 19g; fat 7.1g; cholesterol 86.3mg; sodium 981mg.

Acai Bowl

Prep:

10 mins

Total:

10 mins

Servings:

1

Yield:

1 bowl

Ingredients

1 cup acai berry sorbet

2 tablespoons granola

1 banana

2 teaspoons unsweetened coconut flakes

1 teaspoon honey

4 strawberries, sliced

Directions

1

Place acai sorbet in a bowl and top with a layer of granola. Line strawberries and bananas on granola layer and top with coconut and a drizzle of honey.

Nutrition

Per Serving: 551 calories; protein 4.3g; carbohydrates 107.7g; fat 12.8g; sodium 27.5mg.

Banana Cookies

Prep:

15 mins

Cook:

20 mins

Additional:

15 mins

Total:

50 mins

Servings:

36

Yield:

3 dozen

Ingredients

3 ripe bananas

2 cups rolled oats

⅓ cup vegetable oil

1 teaspoon vanilla extract

1 cup dates, pitted and chopped

Directions

1

Preheat oven to 350 degrees F.

2

In a large bowl, mash the bananas. Stir in oats, dates, oil, and vanilla. Mix well, and allow to sit for 15 minutes. Drop by teaspoonfuls onto an ungreased cookie sheet.

3

Bake for 20 minutes in the preheated oven, or until lightly brown.

Nutrition

Per Serving: 56 calories; protein 0.8g; carbohydrates 8.4g; fat 2.4g; sodium 0.5mg.

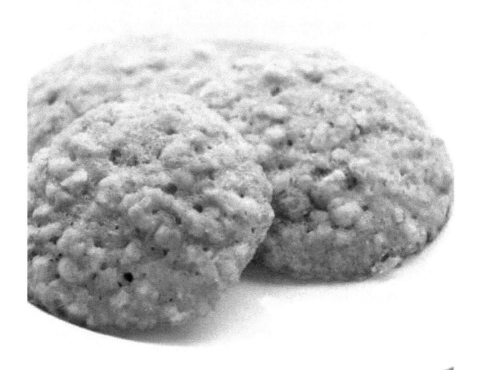

Banana Chips

Prep:

5 mins

Cook:

2 hrs

Total:

2 hrs 5 mins

Servings:

1

Yield:

1 serving

Ingredients

1 firm banana, thinly sliced

Directions

1

Preheat oven to 175 degrees F. Line a baking sheet with parchment.

2

Place banana slices in a single layer on prepared baking sheet.

3

Bake in the preheated oven for 1 hour; turn banana slices over. Continue baking banana slices until dry and crisp, about 1 hour more.

Nutrition

Per Serving: 105 calories; protein 1.3g; carbohydrates 27g; fat 0.4g; sodium 1.2mg.

Coconut Shrimp

Prep:

15 mins

Cook:

15 mins

Total:

30 mins

Servings:

4

Yield:

4 servings

Ingredients

1 pound large shrimp, peeled and deveined

⅓ cup cornstarch

1 teaspoon salt

¾ teaspoon cayenne pepper

2 cups flaked sweetened coconut

3 egg whites, beaten until foamy

Directions

1

Preheat an oven to 400 degrees F (200 degrees C). Lightly coat a baking sheet with cooking spray.

2

Rinse and dry shrimp with paper towels. Mix cornstarch, salt, and cayenne pepper in a shallow bow; pour coconut flakes in a separate shallow bowl. Working with one shrimp at a time, dredge it in the cornstarch mixture, then dip it in the egg white, and roll it in the coconut, making sure to coat the shrimp well. Place on the prepared baking sheet, and repeat with the remaining shrimp.

3

Bake the shrimp until they are bright pink on the outside and the meat is no longer transparent in the center and the coconut is browned, 15 to 20 minutes, flipping the shrimp halfway through.

Nutritions

Per Serving: 310 calories; protein 22.5g; carbohydrates 29.3g; fat 11.4g; cholesterol 172.6mg; sodium 927.7mg.

Tomato Basil Bruschetta

Prep:

20 mins

Cook:

5 mins

Additional:

15 mins

Total:

40 mins

Servings:

10

Yield:

10 servings

Ingredients

2 large tomatoes, diced

½ cup finely chopped red bell pepper

¼ cup finely chopped red onion

¼ cup balsamic vinegar

¼ cup olive oil (Optional)

10 leaves fresh basil, chopped

2 cloves garlic, minced

1 (1 pound) loaf French bread, cut into 1/4-inch slices

¼ cup olive oil (Optional)

¼ cup shredded mozzarella cheese

Directions

1

Combine tomatoes, bell pepper, onion, balsamic vinegar, 1/4 cup olive oil, basil, and garlic; let tomato mixture rest for 15 to 30 minutes.

2

Set oven rack about 6 inches from the heat source and preheat the oven's broiler.

3

Arrange French bread slices on a large baking sheet; drizzle with 1/4 cup olive oil.

4

Toast bread in preheated oven until lightly browned, about 1 minute on each side. Top bread slices with tomato mixture using a slotted spoon, allowing excess liquid to drain. Return bread to baking sheet and sprinkle with mozzarella cheese.

5

Broil in preheated oven until cheese melts, about 3 minutes. Serve immediately.

Nutritions
Per Serving: 248 calories; protein 6.5g; carbohydrates 28.8g; fat 12.2g; cholesterol 1.8mg; sodium 312.8mg.

CHAPTER 5: SMOOTHIES AND DRINKS RECIPES

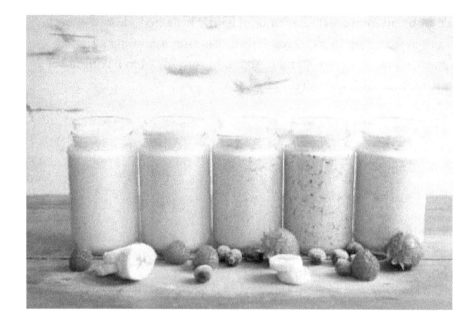

Pineapple Juice

Prep:

5 mins

Total:

5 mins

Servings:

14

Yield:

14 (8 ounce) servings

Ingredients

1 (64 fluid ounce) bottle cranberry juice, chilled

1 (8 ounce) can pineapple tidbits

1 cup cranberries

1 (46 fluid ounce) can pineapple juice

Directions

1

In a punch bowl, combine cranberry juice and pineapple juice. Stir in pineapple tidbits and cranberries. Serve with ice.

Nutrition

Per Serving: 134 calories; protein 0.4g; carbohydrates 33.2g; fat 0.3g; sodium 4.8mg.

Melon Chiller

Prep:

20 mins

Total:

20 mins

Servings:

10

Yield:

10 servings

Ingredients

1 cantaloupe, halved and seeded

2 cups white sugar

ice cubes, as needed

1 gallon water

Directions

1

Scrape the cantaloupe meat lengthwise with a spoon or a melon baller and place in a punch bowl; add the water and sugar. Mix thoroughly until all the sugar is dissolved. Chill with the addition of plenty of ice cubes.

Nutrition

Per Serving: 174 calories; protein 0.5g; carbohydrates 44.5g; fat 0.1g; sodium 20.2mg.

Mexican Chocolate

Prep:

5 mins

Cook:

6 mins

Total:

11 mins

Servings:

8

Yield:

8 servings

Ingredients

1 teaspoon Urfa biber (Turkish chile pepper)

2 tablespoons white sugar

6 cups milk

1 cinnamon stick

1 vanilla bean

8 ounces bittersweet chocolate

½ cup whipped cream

1 tablespoon grated bittersweet chocolate

Directions

1

Split vanilla bean lengthwise with the tip of a sharp knife. Place Urfa biber in a tea infuser.

2

Combine vanilla bean, Urfa biber, milk, and cinnamon stick in a pot.

3

Cook over medium heat, stirring occasionally, until milk is steaming and small bubbles appear, 4 to 5 minutes. Remove Urfa biber. Reduce heat to low. Add chocolate and sugar; stir until chocolate is melted, about 2 minutes. Remove cinnamon stick and vanilla bean.

4

Pour into cups and top with a dollop of whipped cream. Garnish with bittersweet chocolate.

Nutrition

Per Serving: 289 calories; protein 8.2g; carbohydrates 31.3g; fat 14.5g; cholesterol 18.8mg; sodium 81.6mg.

Apple & Carrot Juice

Prep:

10 mins

Total:

10 mins

Servings:

1

Yield:

1 glass

Ingredients

2 stalks celery

1 (1/2 inch) piece fresh ginger

2 apples, quartered

4 carrots, trimmed

Directions

1

Run carrots, apples, and celery through a juicer (alternating carrot, apple, and celery) according to manufacturer's instructions. Add ginger to juicer and process.

Nutrition

Per Serving: 277 calories; protein 4g; carbohydrates 68.6g; fat 1.3g; sodium 265.8mg.

Kale and Spinach Smoothie

Prep:

10 mins

Total:

10 mins

Servings:

1

Yield:

1 serving

Ingredients

2 cups fresh spinach

1 cup almond milk

1 tablespoon peanut butter

1 tablespoon chia seeds (Optional)

1 leaf kale

1 sliced frozen banana

Directions

1

Blend spinach, almond milk, peanut butter, chia seeds, and kale together in a blender until smooth. Add banana and blend until smooth.

Nutritions

Per Serving: 325 calories; protein 10g; carbohydrates 46.1g; fat 13.9g; sodium 293.1mg.

Peanut Butter Strawberry Smoothie

Prep:

10 mins

Total:

10 mins

Servings:

1

Yield:

1 smoothie

Ingredients

8 strawberries, sliced

½ cup plain yogurt

¼ cup milk

2 tablespoons smooth peanut butter

1 teaspoon brown sugar

Directions

1

Blend strawberries, yogurt, milk, peanut butter, and brown sugar together in a blender for 2 minutes; let rest for 10 seconds. Blend until smooth, another 2 minutes.

Nutritions

Per Serving: 363 calories; protein 17.6g; carbohydrates 33.4g; fat 19.9g; cholesterol 12.2mg; sodium 262.8mg.

CHAPTER 6: DESSERTS

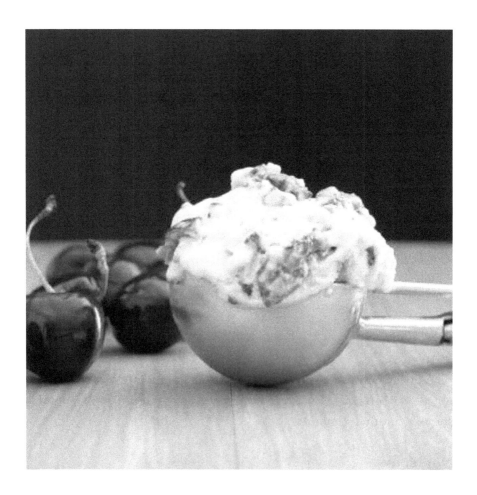

Cherry Frozen Yogurt

Prep:

25 mins

Additional:

4 hrs

Total:

4 hrs 25 mins

Servings:

12

Yield:

6 cups

Ingredients

1 (8 ounce) package cream cheese, softened

1 cup white sugar

1 tablespoon lemon juice

2 cups pitted, chopped fresh cherries

3 cups plain Greek yogurt

Directions

1

In a large bowl, mash the cream cheese with sugar until thoroughly combined; stir in the lemon juice, and mix in the yogurt, about a cup at a time, until the mixture is smooth and creamy. Mix in the cherries. Cover the bowl with plastic wrap, and chill until very cold, at least 4 hours.

2

Pour the mixture into an ice cream freezer, and freeze according to manufacturer's instructions. For firmer texture, pack the frozen yogurt into a covered container, and freeze for several hours.

Nutrition

Per Serving: 212 calories; protein 4.7g; carbohydrates 23.3g; fat 11.7g; cholesterol 31.8mg; sodium 87.8mg

Peach Sorbet

Prep:

10 mins

Cook:

5 mins

Additional:

5 hrs 20 mins

Total:

5 hrs 35 mins

Servings:

8

Yield:

8 servings

Ingredients

2 tablespoons lemon juice

½ cup white sugar

½ cup water

1 pound ripe peaches - peeled, pitted, and chopped

Directions

1

Add peaches to a blender; blend until smooth. Measure out 1 1/2 cups peach puree into a bowl. Immediately stir in lemon juice and refrigerate.

2

Combine water and sugar in a small saucepan and bring to a boil. Stir until sugar is dissolved, about 1 minute. Remove from stove and cool to room temperature. Refrigerate simple syrup until chilled, about 1 hour.

3

Pour chilled peach puree and simple syrup into an ice cream maker and freeze according to manufacturer's instructions, about 20 minutes. Transfer to an airtight container and freeze until firm, about 4 hours.

Nutrition

Per Serving: 60 calories; carbohydrates 15.4g; sodium 2.2mg.

Fresh Strawberries Butter

Prep:

5 mins

Total:

5 mins

Servings:

16

Yield:

16 servings

Ingredients

1 cup confectioners' sugar
1 cup butter, softened
10 ounces hulled strawberries

Directions

1

Combine strawberries, butter, and confectioners' sugar in a blender; blend until smooth.

Nutrition

Per Serving: 138 calories; protein 0.2g; carbohydrates 9.2g; fat 11.6g; cholesterol 30.5mg; sodium 82mg

Mocha Cream

Servings:

16

Yield:

4 cups

Ingredients

2 cups heavy whipping cream
1 tablespoon boiling water
2 tablespoons white sugar
1 tablespoon instant coffee powder

Directions

1

Beat whipping cream and sugar together in mixing bowl until stiff.
Dissolve coffee granules in boiling water. Cool. Add to whipped cream
and beat in. Makes enough to frost and fill one 8 or 9 inch 2 layer
cake. Keep Mocha Cream refrigerated.

Nutrition

Per Serving: 109 calories; protein 0.6g; carbohydrates 2.5g; fat 11g;
cholesterol 40.8mg; sodium 11.4mg.

Peach Tarts

Prep:

15 mins

Cook:

55 mins

Additional:

2 hrs 15 mins

Total:

3 hrs 25 mins

Servings:

10

Yield:

1 9-inch tart

Ingredients

Crust:

1 ⅓ cups all-purpose flour

½ cup unsalted butter, melted

¼ cup white sugar

¼ teaspoon salt

⅛ teaspoon ground nutmeg

⅛ teaspoon ground cardamom

½ teaspoon ground cinnamon

1 teaspoon vanilla extract

Filling:

1 ½ cups fresh blueberries

2 ½ tablespoons honey

2 ½ cups peeled and sliced fresh peaches

1 ½ teaspoons lemon juice

Streusel Topping:

¼ cup all-purpose flour

¼ cup rolled oats

¼ teaspoon ground cinnamon

⅛ teaspoon ground nutmeg

¼ cup firmly packed dark brown sugar

1 pinch salt

½ teaspoon vanilla extract

3 tablespoons unsalted butter, melted

Directions

1

Preheat the oven to 350 degrees F. Lightly grease a 9-inch tart pan with a removable bottom.

2

Mix flour, sugar, cinnamon, salt, nutmeg, and cardamom in a bowl for the crust. Add in melted butter and vanilla extract. Stir until mixture comes together into a soft dough.

3

Place dough in the prepared pan; press evenly over the bottom and up the sides. Use a fork to gently prick the bottom of the crust several times. Place the pan on a baking sheet.

4

Bake in the preheated oven until crust is just beginning to brown, 15 to 20 minutes. Remove from the oven and allow to cool.

5

Toss sliced peaches, blueberries, honey, and lemon juice together in a bowl until evenly coated. Pour filling into the cooled crust, slightly mounding the fruit in the middle.

6

Mix flour, oats, brown sugar, cinnamon, nutmeg, and salt in a bowl until topping is combined. Stir in melted butter and vanilla extract until mixture resembles coarse crumbs. Sprinkle topping evenly over the filling.

7

Return the tart to the oven and bake until topping is lightly browned and filling is bubbling, 38 to 42 minutes. Cool to room temperature before removing from the pan. Place tart in the refrigerator and cool completely before slicing.

Nutrition

Per Serving: 271 calories; protein 2.7g; carbohydrates 36.7g; fat 13.1g; cholesterol 33.6mg; sodium 79.2mg.

Apple Compote

Prep:

10 mins

Cook:

10 mins

Total:

20 mins

Servings:

10

Yield:

10 servings

Ingredients

¼ cup unsalted butter

½ cup pecans

3 Granny Smith apples - peeled, cored, and chopped

2 tablespoons white sugar

water

½ cup golden raisins

1 pinch salt

1 tablespoon whiskey (Optional)

1 teaspoon vanilla extract

Directions

1

Melt butter in a saucepan over medium heat; cook and stir pecans in melted butter until lightly toasted, 2 to 3 minutes. Transfer toasted pecans to a bowl with a slotted spoon, reserving butter in pan. Cook and stir apples in reserved butter until apples begin to soften, about 2 minutes; add sugar.

2

Stir water, raisins, and salt into apple mixture. Simmer, stirring occasionally, until raisins are plump, about 5 minutes. Add whiskey, vanilla extract, and toasted pecans.

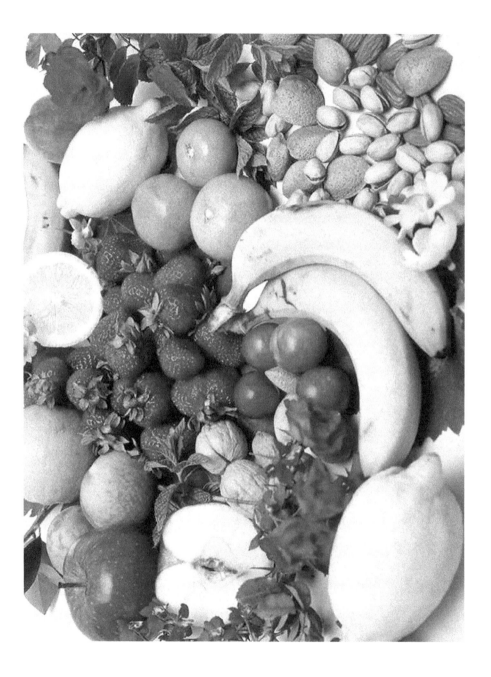